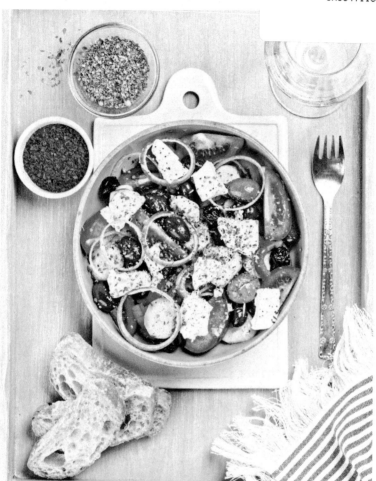

THE GESTATIONAL DIABETES

COOKBOOK

A GESTATIONAL DIABETES DISEASE DIET GUIDE

By
Selena Sablon RD
Copyright © by Wentworth Publishing House

Published by
Savour Press, a DBA of Wentworth Publishing House

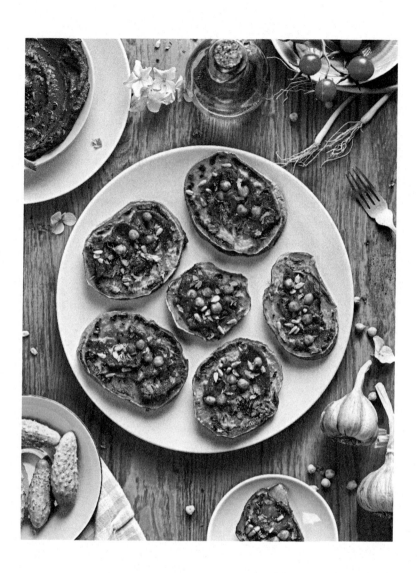

Let's get it started!

Welcome to Savour. Food is one of man's basic needs, which we need fulfill each day. But sometimes, some foods may bring harm to your body, particularly if taken more than your recommended daily allowance. There are foods that can fill our body with nutrients, but still too much of them can make you overweight and sick. Which brings us to the purpose behind why we created this Gestational Diabetes Diet cookbook, believing that this can help you in your healthy living. We stand by our philosophy that you can create a wholesome life, away from sickness and pain with our recipes that we write, so every bit of it will become a part of your daily mantra. We don't want to scare you, instead we are here to inspire you, by guiding you with our best selection of recipes to stay fit or achieve that wow figure that you desire. Don't miss every recipe as they are all helpful in your goal to stay healthy.

About This Book

You may have gotten the news recently from your doctor and may have even read up about it online which is how to manage and treat gestational diabetes. Well, *Savour* is here to open your mind about the goodness that this Gestational diabetes diet brings to your health and with our recipes, we are sure you will embrace this diet program feeling satisfied. It opens with Garlic Rosemary Pork Chops, and followed by several beef recipes like Taco Cups, Burger Fat Bombs, and then some shrimp recipes, chicken, fish and a lot more. Most of the recipes require you to combine all ingredients after sautéing the fish or beef, in one sitting and let the oven finish the job. Most of our ingredients call for cheese, butter, beef, chicken, salmon, mahi-mahi, shrimp, bacon, eggs, and avocados, low-carb vegetables like spinach, zucchini, butternut squash, Butterhead lettuce, asparagus, and artichoke. They also call for olive or vegetable oil for frying and no flour from wheat, corn and rice, but there is one recipe that requires you to use almond flour. Let's get ready to have a fun time!

6 Common Conversions You Need to Know

1 tablespoon = 3 teaspoons

4 tablespoons = 1/4 cup

1 cup = 250 mL

1 pint = 500 mL

1 quart = 0.95 L

1 gallon = 3.8 L

Common Weight Conversions

1 ounce = 28 g

4 ounces or 1/4 pound =113 g

1/3 pound=150 g

8 ounces or 1/2 pound =230 g

2/3 pound =300 g

12 ounces or 3/4 pound =340 g

1 pound or 16 ounces =450 g

2 pounds= 900 g

Common Metric Conversions

1 teaspoon = 5 mL

1 tablespoon or 1/2 fluid ounce =15 mL

1 fluid ounce or 1/8 cup= 30 mL

1/4 cup or 2 fluid ounces =60 mL

1/3 cup= 80 mL

1/2 cup or 4 fluid ounces=120 mL

2/3 cup=160 mL

3/4 cup or 6 fluid ounces=180 mL

1 cup or 8 fluid ounces or half a pint= 240 mL

2 cups or 1 pint or 16 fluid ounces =475 mL

4 cups or 2 pints or 1 quart = 950 mL

4 quarts or 1 gallon = 3.8 L

INTRODUCTION

When it comes to eating healthier low carbohydrate recipes are highly recommended, but if you think you can't live without rice or carbohydrates because the food will not nearly be as tasty, we are to tell you the results are well worth the short-term inconvenience. So, why not give yourself a chance by trying our curated recipes designed to combat and reverse diabetes. Our recipes are categorized into pork, beef, chicken, fish, shrimp, and bacon. We are pretty sure you will like the recipes that have been prepared in this cookbook with the guide of physician Aqsa Layla MD and you will find them to be delicious and nutritious. They are simple, and the instructions are succinct with few ingredients. You are not required to prepare tacos or pasta, but use avocado, pepper, Butterhead lettuce or cheese as your taco shell. Instead of using Pappardelle for your pasta, you can use zucchini by cutting it into long flat strips or spiralized it to form into corkscrew pasta. Just look in our recipes and you will be surprised at their unique presentation.

OVERVIEW

Diabetes is a hormonal disorder, which results in high blood glucose levels. Glucose is the driving fuel of our body. Everything we eat is finally broken down into glucose which is utilized by the cells to gain energy. This glucose is supplied to the body organs through blood. The excess is either discarded or stored in the body in some other form. There must be a certain balance of blood glucose to facilitate its better use. If the glucose level is too high, it can lead to numbness or even retardation. Or if it is too low, it can lead to hypoglycemia. This balance of glucose is maintained through two hormones named Insulin and Glucagon. Glycogen allows the glucose to be released into the blood whereas Insulin does the opposite, i.e., a decrease in the blood glucose levels. In diabetes, the pancreatic cells producing the Insulin hormone are affected, and they reduce the Insulin production. This led to the increase of glucose in the blood to a harmful level.

Ideally, a person should have 70 to 130 mg/dL glucose in the blood. If the amount increases and persists in the high range, the person will then be suffering from diabetes. Once the beta cells in the pancreas are damaged, they do not repair easily.

Gestational diabetes (GDM)

As the name indicates, this type of diabetes can occur to a mother during the gestational period or pregnancy. The good news is that it is not permanent but a temporary condition and persists only during the pregnancy. It is caused by the production of certain hormones from the placenta of the baby, and these hormones can disrupt the functioning of the insulin. Therefore, the body becomes insulin resistant. It is not always harmful, but the condition can get critical in case of malnutrition or poor dietary intake. Which is why we have created this cookbook to help you or a loved one manage and treat gestational diabetes.

Incorporate Foods That Promote Insulin Sensitivity

There are certain food sources and drinks that might be advantageous for gestational diabetes:

- Monounsaturated fats: Research proposes that eating foods high in monounsaturated unsaturated fats like olive oil, avocados and nuts may advance fat loss in the liver.

- Whey protein: Whey protein has been shown to diminish liver fat by up to 20% in overweight women. What's more, it might help lower liver compound levels and furnish different advantages in individuals with further developed liver sickness.

- Green tea: One investigation found that cell reinforcements in green tea called catechins helped decline liver fat and aggravation in individuals with NAFLD.

- Solvent fiber: Some examination proposes that eating 10–14 grams of dissolvable fiber every day may help diminish liver fat, decline liver compound levels and increase insulin sensitivity.

CONTENTS

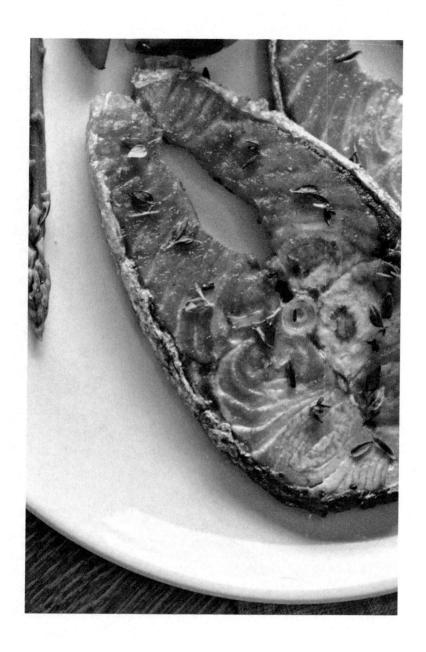

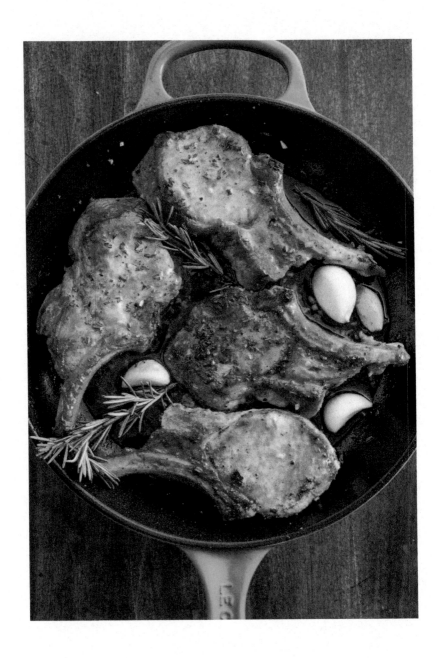

Pork

Garlic Rosemary Pork Chops

Weeknight dinner is getting more exciting as your family knows well how delicious these garlicky-herbed pork chops are. The pork chops are tender-juicy by searing them and brushed with garlic butter. Serve baked pork chops with garlic butter.

Servings: 4

Ingredients

4 pieces **pork loin chops**

Dash of freshly **ground black pepper**

Pinch of **Kosher salt**

2 minced **cloves garlic**

1 tablespoon freshly minced **rosemary**

1 tablespoon **extra-virgin olive oil**

1/2 cup (1 stick) melted **butter**

DIRECTIONS:

Preheat oven at 375° F.

Rub pork loin chops with a pinch of salt and a dash of pepper.

Combine in a small bowl the garlic, rosemary and butter, set aside.

Heat olive oil in an oven safe skillet on moderate heat.

Cook pork chops by searing for four minutes until golden brown. Flip once and cook for another 4 minutes.

Brush browned pork chops with a generous amount of garlic butter.

Place the skillet in preheated oven and cook the pork chops for ten to twelve minutes until warmed through.

Serve pork chops with extra garlic butter.

Enjoy!

Nutritional Information: 494 calorie; 46.4 g fat (22.5 g saturated fat); 130 mg cholesterol; 258 mg sodium; 1.1 g carbohydrate; 0.4 g dietary fiber; 0 g total sugars; 18.4 g protein.

BEEF

BLT BURGERS

Be a bit creative when preparing burgers to make it more appealing to your kids who dislike vegetables. Turn bacon slices into weaves and place below the burger with bacon weaves, top with herb mayo, then the burger, lettuce, tomato and top with bacon weave.

Servings: 4

Ingredients

1 pound **ground beef**

1 pound **bacon slices**, halved

Fresh **ground black pepper**

Kosher salt

Juice of 1/2 lemon

1/2 cup **mayonnaise**

Butterhead lettuce, for serving

3 tablespoons finely chopped **chives**

2 sliced **tomatoes**

Directions

Preheat oven at 400 degrees F. Prepare a baking rack by placing it inside of your baking sheet, set aside.

Prepare the bacon weaves by placing three bacon halves on a baking rack side by side.

Lift 1 end of the bacon slice in the middle.

19

Place the 4th bacon half on top of the slices on the sides and below the slice in the middle.

Place the slice in the middle going back down. Pull upwards the 2 side bacon strips and put the fifth bacon half over the middle bacon piece and below the sides.

Place the side bacon slices back down.

Pull upward the other end of the middle bacon slice and put the sixth bacon slice over the side bacon pieces and below the middle bacon slice.

Follow these steps for the second bacon weave. Season the bacon weave with pepper; bake for twenty-five minutes until crisp-tender and drain on paper towel. Let bacon cool for ten minutes.

Make the burgers:

Preheat a grill or grill pan on medium-high heat. Form the ground beef into large equal size of patties; season each side with a pinch of salt and black pepper. Place in grill and cook for four minutes each side for medium doneness.

Make herb mayo:

Whisk in a small bowl the lemon juice, mayonnaise and chives, set aside.

Assemble burgers:

Place the bottom of each burger with bacon weave and spread with herb mayo. Place on top of mayo the burger, Butterhead lettuce, tomato slices and the remaining bacon weave.

Serve!

Nutritional Information: 911 calorie; 65.7 g fat (20.3 g saturated fat); 230 mg cholesterol; 2677 mg sodium; 11.1 g carbohydrate; 1.5 g dietary fiber; 4.1 g total sugars; 68.3 g protein.

CHILI

This Keto-inspired chili recipe is enough to keep you going. It is loaded with myriads of seasonings, spices, greens and toppings, so nothing to worry if you are concerned about your health. Drain the fried bacon and the sautéed ground beef before you mix them with the vegetables.

Servings: 8

Ingredients

3 slices of **bacon** (cut into ½-inch strips)

2 chopped **celery stalks**

1/4 chopped medium **yellow onion**

1/2 cup sliced **baby Bellas**

1 chopped **green bell pepper**

2 pounds **ground beef**

2 minced **cloves garlic**

2 teaspoons **ground cumin**

2 tablespoons **chili powder**

2 tablespoons **smoked paprika**

2 teaspoons **dried oregano**

Kosher salt

Freshly **ground black pepper**

2 cups **low-sodium beef broth**

For garnish:

Shredded **cheddar**

Sour cream

Sliced **green onions**

Sliced **avocado**

Directions

Cook bacon in a large pot on moderate heat until crisp. Remove from pot immediately using a slotted spoon and drain on paper towel.

Stir-fry the onion, mushrooms, celery and pepper in the same pot and cook for six minutes until the vegetables are cooked.

Stir in garlic and cook for 1 minute until fragrant.

Push the veggies to the side of pan and place the beef in the center.

Stir and cook until there is no more pink color in the beef. Drain excess fat from beef and return pan to the heat.

Pour the paprika, oregano, cumin, chili powder, salt and pepper into the beef mixture, stirring often and cook for two minutes.

Pour the broth and simmer; cook for ten to fifteen minutes until the broth is almost dried.

Spoon the chili into individual bowls.

Garnish with sour cream, bacon crisps, shredded cheese, avocado slices and green onions.

Serve!

Nutritional Information: 276 calorie; 10.8 g fat (3.8 g saturated fat); 109 mg cholesterol; 396 mg sodium; 4.5 g carbohydrate; 1.9 g dietary fiber; 1.3 g total sugars; 38.7 g protein.

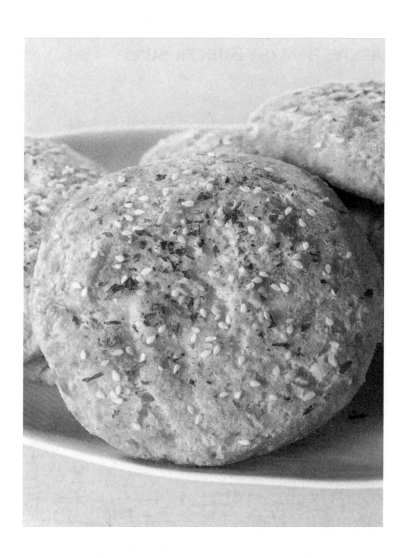

DIABETES HEALTHY BURGER BUNS

If you are looking for a diabetic friendly bun for your burger, this recipe is what you are looking for. These creamy and cheesy buns are sugar-free, so it is safe for your health. The top part of the buns is drizzled with sesame seeds and parsley for a nutty and crunchy texture.

Servings: 6

Ingredients

4 ounces **cream cheese**

2 cups shredded **mozzarella**

3 cups **almond flour**

3 large **eggs**

1 teaspoon **kosher salt**

2 teaspoons **baking powder**

4 tablespoons melted **butter**

Dried parsley

Sesame seeds

Directions

Preheat oven at 400° Fahrenheit and line a large baking sheet with a parchment paper.

Melt in a large microwave-safe bowl the cream cheese and mozzarella cheese.

Stir in eggs and add the almond flour, salt and baking powder.

26

Shape the dough into six ball pieces, slightly flatten out and place them on the baking sheet.

Brush dough with melted butter and garnish with parsley and sesame seeds.

Bake for ten to twelve minutes until golden.

Enjoy!

Nutritional Information: 291 calorie; 25.8 g fat (11.4 g saturated fat); 139 mg cholesterol; 597 mg sodium; 5.2 g carbohydrate; 1.7 g dietary fiber; 0.2 g total sugars;10.6 g protein.

Taco Cups

Prepare taco cups without using flour while you are following gestational diabetes diet. This time use baked melted cheese as your taco cups by placing them on the bottom of muffin tin as molders, and then fill with spicy and garlicky beef mixture, topped with avocado, cilantro, tomatoes, and sour cream.

Servings: 8

Ingredients

1 pound **ground beef**

1 tablespoon **extra-virgin olive oil**

3 1/2 cups **shredded cheddar**

3 minced **cloves garlic**

1 chopped **onion**

1/2 teaspoon **ground cumin**

1 teaspoon **chili powder**

Kosher salt

1/2 teaspoon **paprika**

Freshly **ground black pepper**

For serving:

Diced **avocado**

Sour cream

Chopped **cilantro**

Chopped **tomatoes**

Directions

Preheat oven at 375° Fahrenheit.

Prepare a large baking sheet by lining the bottom with parchment paper.

Spoon two tablespoons of cheese onto the baking sheet, at least 2 inches apart; bake for six minutes until the edges are turning golden and bubbly. Let cheese cool on sheet for 1 to 2 minutes.

Coat the bottom of a muffin tin with cooking spray. Slowly remove the melted cheese slices with pancake turner and neatly place on the tin's bottom. Let stand for ten minutes.

Heat olive oil in a large skillet on medium heat and sauté the onion for five minutes until soft.

Stir-fry the garlic and ground beef; crumble with a wooden spoon; cook for six minutes until brown; drain.

Sprinkle the meat with salt, pepper, paprika, cumin and chili powder.

Place cheese cups into a serving plate and fill each with beef mixture.

Garnish with sour cream, diced avocado, chopped cilantro and chopped tomatoes.

Enjoy!

Nutritional Information: 215 calorie; 8.9 g fat (3.7 g saturated fat); 61 mg cholesterol; 364 mg sodium; 2.9 g carbohydrate; 0.5 g dietary fiber; 0.9 g total sugars; 29.5 g protein.

ICEBURGERS

A great way to enjoy burgers with less carbohydrate is to use iceberg lettuce as your bun. Top the sliced lettuce head with cheddar and place on top with cheeseburger, bacon slice, tomato slice, ranch dressing and cover with another lettuce head slice.

Servings: 4

Ingredients

4 slices **bacon**

1 large head **iceberg lettuce**

1 pound **ground beef**

Pinch of **kosher salt**

1 sliced red **onion**

Dash of freshly **ground black pepper**

1 sliced **tomato**

4 slices **cheddar**

For serving:

Ranch dressing

Directions

Create buns by slicing eight large rounds from the tip of the head of iceberg lettuce.

Cook the bacon in a large pan on moderate heat until crispy and drain on plate lined with paper towel.

Sauté the onion slices in the bacon fat for three minutes each side until tender, set aside. Wipe out skillet and reheat on medium high heat.

Form the ground beef into four large burger patties and sprinkle each side with salt and pepper.

Cook beef in hot oil for four minutes each side for medium doneness.

Place one slice of cheddar on top of each lettuce burger and cover the pan. Cook for 1 minute until the cheese has melted; remove burger from heat.

To assemble burger:

Place on top of iceberg lettuce round with cheeseburger, and then one bacon slice, then tomato slice and drizzle with dressing. Finally, place the second iceberg lettuce round on top.

Place a toothpick to hold on to the filling. Repeat the steps with the rest of the iceberg lettuce round, cheeseburger, bacon slice, tomato slice, ranch dressing and second iceberg lettuce round.

Serve!

Nutritional Information: 404 calories; 17.4 g fat (6.5 g saturated fat); 128 mg cholesterol; 778 mg sodium; 10.1 g carbohydrate; 2 g dietary fiber; 3.8 g total sugars; 49.7 g protein.

TACO STUFFED AVOCADOS

Use your creativity when it comes to preparing Keto recipe, and if you like taco, try using avocado instead of carbohydrate loaded tortilla. Remove some flesh of avocado and fill it with browned meat, avocado flesh, cheese, lettuce, grape tomato and a dollop of sour cream.

Servings: 4-8

Ingredients

4 ripe **avocados**

1 tablespoon **extra-virgin olive oil**

Juice of 1 lime

1 pound **ground beef**

1 chopped medium **onion**

Kosher salt

1 packet **taco seasoning**

Freshly **ground black pepper**

1/2 cup **shredded lettuce**

2/3 cups **shredded Mexican cheese**

1/2 cup quartered **grape tomatoes**

Topping:

Sour cream

Directions

Cut the avocado into half and remove the pit. Scoop out flesh of avocado to create a large well. Dice the flesh, set aside.

Squeeze out lime juice all over the avocados to prevent browning.

Heat olive oil in a medium-size pan on moderate heat. Sauté the onion and stir for five minutes until tender.

Stir in ground beef, and crumble in taco seasoning using a wooden spoon. Sprinkle with salt and pepper.

Cook for six minutes until the meat is browned. Remove pan from heat and drain excess fat.

Stuff avocado half with beef mixture and garnish with avocado flesh, Mexican cheese, shredded lettuce, grape tomato and sour cream dollop.

Enjoy!

Nutritional Information: 816 calorie; 63.4 g fat (19.9 g saturated fat); 131 mg cholesterol; 285 mg sodium; 24.2 g carbohydrate; 14.2 g dietary fiber; 3.4 g total sugars; 42.1 g protein.

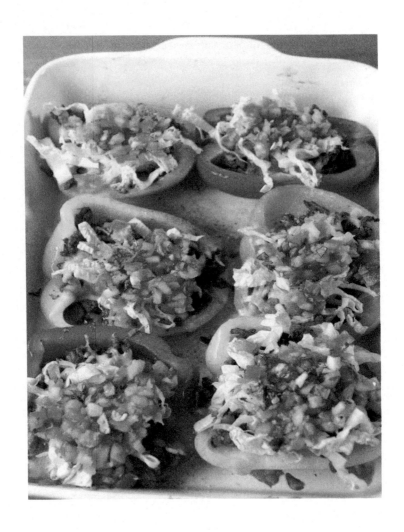

TACO STUFFED PEPPERS

Give a twist to your taco by filling the bell pepper halves with sautéed ground beef cooked with herbs and spices. Oil the peppers before stuffing the meat mixture and cheese. Bake the peppers, garnish taco with lettuce.

Servings: 6

Ingredients

1 pound **ground beef**

Extra-virgin olive oil

1 minced **clove garlic**

1/2 chopped **onion**

Freshly **ground black pepper**

Kosher salt

1 teaspoon **chili powder**

2 tablespoons chopped **cilantro**

1/2 teaspoon **smoked paprika**

1/2 teaspoon **ground cumin**

1 cup shredded **cheddar**

3 **bell peppers**

1 cup shredded **lettuce**

1 cup shredded **Monterey Jack**

For serving:

Hot sauce

Lime wedges

Pico de Gallo

Directions

Remove seeds of peppers and cut into half.

Preheat oven at 375° and coat a large baking dish with cooking spray.

Heat 1 tablespoon of extra-virgin olive oil in a large skillet on medium heat.

Sauté the onion and cook for five minutes until tender. Add the garlic and stir-fry until aromatic for 1 minute longer.

Add beef and stir-fry for five minutes until the pinkish color is gone, drain excess fat.

Stir in ground cumin, paprika and chili powder and sprinkle with salt and pepper.

Drizzle the bell peppers with olive oil; season bell peppers with salt and pepper. Neatly place the bell peppers with cut side up on the baking dish.

Stuff each pepper with meat mixture.

Sprinkle stuffed pepper with cheese, bake for twenty minutes until tender-crisp and the cheese melts.

Place on top with shredded lettuce. Serve with hot sauce, Pico de Gallo and lime wedges.

Enjoy!

Nutritional Information: 244 calorie; 10.2 g fat (3.8 g saturated fat); 77 mg cholesterol; 282 mg sodium; 8.1 g carbohydrate; 1.6 g dietary fiber; 4 g total sugars; 29.7 g protein.

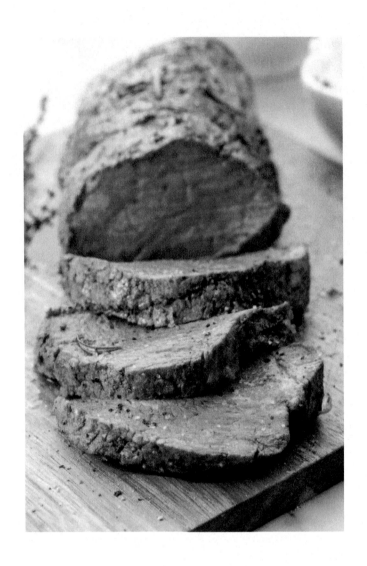

BEEF TENDERLOIN

Enjoy every bite of this tender-juicy beef with yogurt sauce made of lemon, horseradish, Greek yogurt and sour cream. Marinate the beef in a mixture of mustard, olive oil, vinegar, herbs, honey, bay leaf and spices for several hours and season with rosemary, garlic, salt and pepper before roasting in oven.

Servings: 4

Ingredients

For beef:

2 pounds **beef tenderloin**

1/2 cup **extra-virgin olive oil**

2 tablespoons **whole grain mustard**

2 tablespoons **balsamic vinegar**

3 sprigs **fresh rosemary**

3 sprigs **fresh thyme**

1 **bay leaf**

2 tablespoons **honey**

2 crushed **cloves garlic**

1 teaspoon freshly **ground black pepper**

1 teaspoon **kosher salt**

1 minced **clove garlic**

1 teaspoon **dried rosemary**

For yogurt sauce:

1/4 cup **sour cream**

1/2 cup **Greek yogurt**

Juice of 1/2 lemon

1 teaspoon **prepared horseradish**

Kosher salt

Directions

Combine in a large bowl the olive oil, mustard, vinegar, thyme, bay leaf, garlic, honey, and rosemary.

In a large bowl, mix together oil, balsamic vinegar, mustard, thyme, rosemary, bay leaf, crushed garlic, and honey; marinate the meat with cover for 1 hour or overnight in refrigerator.

Preheat oven at 450 degrees F.

Prepare a rimmed baking sheet and line with aluminum foil; and then insert a wire rack. Remove beef tenderloin from marinade.

Pat the beef dry with paper towels and season with minced garlic, rosemary, salt and pepper.

Place beef on the wire rack, roast for twenty minutes until done, depending on your desired doneness.

Let rest for five to ten minutes before slicing.

Meanwhile, combine in a bowl the yogurt sauce ingredients. Serve tenderloin with sauce.

Enjoy!

Nutritional Information: 890 calorie; 50.4 g fat (14.6 g saturated fat); 219 mg cholesterol; 881 mg sodium; 21.6 g carbohydrate; 0.9 g dietary fiber; 17.2 g total sugars; 86.5 g protein.

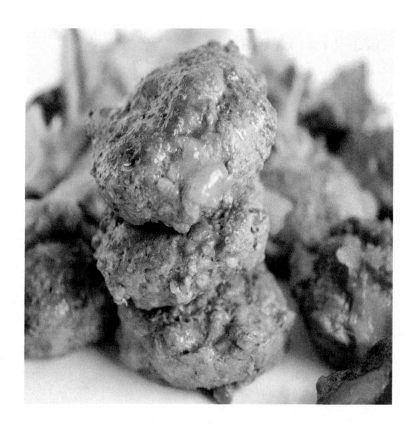

41

Burger Fat Bombs

Let your guests taste these lovely burgers, which is simply made by seasoning the ground beef with salt, garlic powder and black pepper, and spoon 1 tablespoon of beef into the muffin tin, topping it in this sequence: 1 piece butter, beef, 1 piece cheese and 1 tablespoon beef and bake the burger.

Servings: 20

Ingredients

Cooking spray

1 pound **ground beef**

Kosher salt

1/2 teaspoon **garlic powder**

2 tablespoons **cold butter** (cut into 20 pieces)

Freshly **ground black pepper**

1/4 (8 ounces) **block cheddar cheese** (cut into 20 pieces)

For serving:

Lettuce leaves

Thinly sliced **tomatoes**

Mustard

Directions

Preheat oven at 375° F.

Prepare a mini muffin tin by greasing with cooking spray.

Combine in a medium-sized bowl the beef with salt, pepper and garlic powder.

Spoon 1 tablespoon of beef mixture and press into the bottom of muffin tin cup.

Put one piece of butter on top of meat and then press 1 tablespoon of beef mixture on top of butter.

Put on top of meat one piece of cheese and put another beef on top of cheese to cover.

Do these steps for the rest of beef, butter, beef, cheese, and beef for the rest of muffin tin cups.

Bake for fifteen minutes until the meat is no longer pinkish in color, let cool slightly before removing from tin with a metal offset spatula.

Serve Keto burgers with lettuce leaves, ripe tomatoes and mustard.

Enjoy!

Nutritional Information: 99 calorie; 6.2 g fat (3.3 g saturated fat); 35 mg cholesterol; 104 mg sodium; 0.9 g carbohydrate; 0.2 g dietary fiber; 0.2 g total sugars; 9.8 g protein

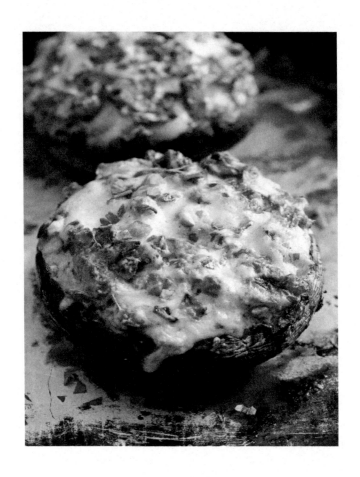

PHILLY CHEESESTEAK STUFFED PORTOBELLOS

Each beef stuffed portobello mushroom is expected to be wiped out once serve on your dining table. The secret is the cheesy taste of provolone and peppery flavor from the bell peppers. This recipe does not use seasonings to enhance the flavors; but the right timing of blended ingredients bring its natural flavor.

Servings: 4

Ingredients

1 pound **sirloin**

4 medium **portobello mushrooms**

3 tablespoons **extra-virgin olive oil**, divided

2 sliced **bell peppers**

1 sliced into half-moons **onion**

Freshly **ground black pepper**

Pinch of **kosher salt**

4 slices **provolone**

Chopped **parsley**

Directions

Remove stems and gills of portobello mushrooms, set aside.

Preheat oven at 350° F.

Place in a large baking sheet the mushrooms and brush the caps with one tablespoon of olive oil.

Season the mushroom with salt and pepper and place with stem side-up.

Heat one tablespoon of olive oil in a large pan. Stir-fry the onions and peppers; season with salt and pepper.

Cook for five minutes until the veggies are tender-crisp, remove immediately from heat.

Pour the remaining 2 tablespoons of olive oil and heat over medium-high. Rub the sirloin with salt and pepper and cook for three minutes until each side are seared.

Turn off stove heat and place the cooked vegetables in the pan, toss to combine with the steak.

Fill each mushroom cap with steak mixture and top with provolone. Bake the mushrooms for twenty minutes until provolone is melty and the peppers are tender-crisp.

Spread on top with parsley. Serve immediately.

Enjoy!

Nutritional Information: 450 calorie; 25.2 g fat (9 g saturated fat); 121 mg cholesterol; 363 mg sodium; 10.9 g carbohydrate; 2.5 g dietary fiber; 45.5 g protein; 4.4 g total sugars.

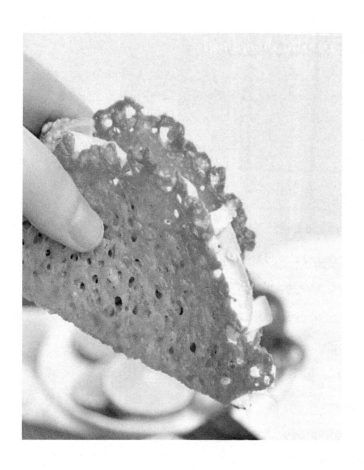

CHEESE TACO SHELLS

Transform cheese into taco shells by baking and stuff with beef mixture cooked with taco seasonings. Each cheese taco is garnished with lettuce, tomatoes, and hot sauce for added flavor and extra crunchiness.

Servings: 4

Ingredients

1 pound **ground beef**

2 cups shredded **cheddar**

1 tablespoons **vegetable oil**

Freshly **ground black pepper**

1 tablespoon **taco seasoning**

1 chopped **white onion**

For serving:

Chopped **tomatoes**

Shredded **lettuce**

Hot sauce

Directions

Preheat oven at 375 degrees F. Place parchment paper on the baking sheet and spray on top with cooking spray.

Spoon about ½ cup of cheddar mound and place on the baking sheet; season with pepper.

Bake until the cheese is becoming melty and a bit crispy for five to seven minutes.

Place on paper towel to remove excess oil.

Turn upside down two drinking glasses and connect the two glasses with a wooden spoon to resemble like a bridge.

With a spatula, hang the cheese mounds on the wooden spoon to create taco shells. Let cool.

Heat the vegetable oil in a large skillet on moderate heat. Cook the onions for five minutes until soft and stir in ground beef until brownish for six minutes longer.

Drain excess fats. Stir in taco seasoning.

To assemble, fill each cheese taco with sautéed beef and garnish with shredded lettuce and chopped tomatoes.

Serve with hot sauce.

Enjoy!

Nutritional Information: 365 calorie; 14.5 g fat (5.8 g saturated fat); 113 mg cholesterol; 686 mg sodium; 6.9 g carbohydrate; 1 g dietary fiber; 2.8 g total sugars; 48.7 g protein.

No Carb Philly Cheesesteaks

This no carb recipe is what you need if you are following the Keto Diet plan. Fill lettuce leaves with cheesy steak mixture, which is a combination of sautéed vegetables, spices, provolone and skirt steak. Garnish each lettuce cup with parsley for extra crunchiness.

Servings: 4

Ingredients

1 thinly sliced large **onion**

2 tablespoons **vegetable oil**, divided

1 teaspoon dried **oregano**

2 thinly sliced large **bell peppers**

Freshly **ground black pepper**

Kosher salt

1 cup **shredded provolone**

1 pound thinly sliced **skirt steak**

8 large **Butterhead lettuce leaves**

1 tablespoon **parsley**, chopped

Directions

Heat one tablespoon of vegetable oil in a large pan on moderate heat.

Stir-fry the onion and bell pepper; season with salt, pepper and oregano.

Cook for five minutes until the vegetables are tender. Remove the onions and peppers from pan.

Stir-fry the skirt steak in a single layer and sprinkle with a pinch of salt and dash of pepper.

Cook the steak until one side is seared for two minutes, flipping to sear the other side for two minutes.

Return the onion mixture to the pan, toss to coat well with steak.

Sprinkle shredded provolone on top of the onions and steak, cover and cook for 1 minute until the cheese is melty.

Remove steak mixture from heat. Place lettuce leaves on a large plate and fill each one with steak mixture.

Garnish on top with parsley.

Enjoy!

Nutritional Information: 448 calorie; 27.3 g fat (11.4 g saturated fat); 90 mg cholesterol; 9.7 g carbohydrate; 419 mg sodium; 2.1 g dietary fiber; 5.1 g total sugars; 40.2 g protein.

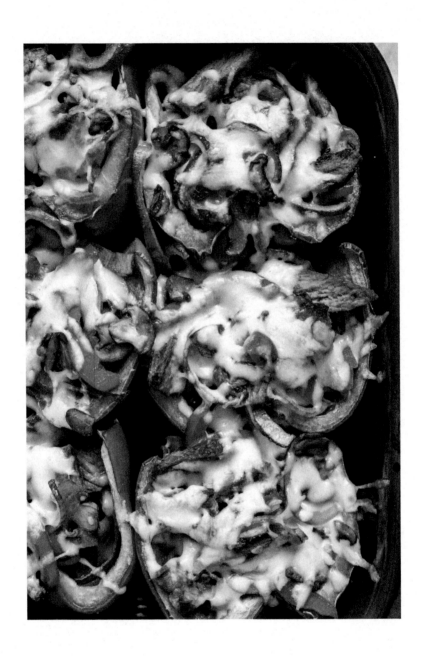

CHEESESTEAK STUFFED PEPPERS

These delightful stuffed peppers is given a twist by lining the bottom of baked bell pepper halves with provolone and topped with steak mixture and finally cover the top with another piece of provolone before broiling. The meat mixture is a blend of cremini mushrooms, Italian seasoning and spices.

Servings: 4

Ingredients

1 tablespoon **vegetable oil**

4 **bell peppers** cut into halve

1 sliced large **onion**

Kosher salt

16 ounces sliced **cremini mushrooms**

Freshly **ground black pepper**

2 teaspoons **Italian seasoning**

1 1/2 pounds thinly sliced **sirloin steak**

16 slices **provolone**

For garnish:

Freshly chopped **parsley**

Directions

Preheat oven at 325 degree Fahrenheit. Lay bell pepper halves with cut-side up in a large baking dish. Bake for half an hour until tender.

Heat vegetable oil in a large pan on moderate high heat and sauté the onions and mushroom.

53

Season mushroom with salt and pepper; cook for six minutes until soft.

Add the sirloin steak and add salt and pepper if desired. Cook steak mixture for three minutes and stir in Italian seasoning.

Place provolone on the bottom of peppers.

Place on top of provolone the steak mixture and then cover with provolone.

Broil stuffed peppers for three minutes until golden.

Garnish peppers with parsley.

Serve!

Nutritional Information: 831 calorie; 45 g fat (23.9 g saturated fat; 231 mg cholesterol; 1145 mg sodium; 20 g carbohydrate; 3.2 g dietary fiber; 10.4 g total sugars; 84.8 g protein.

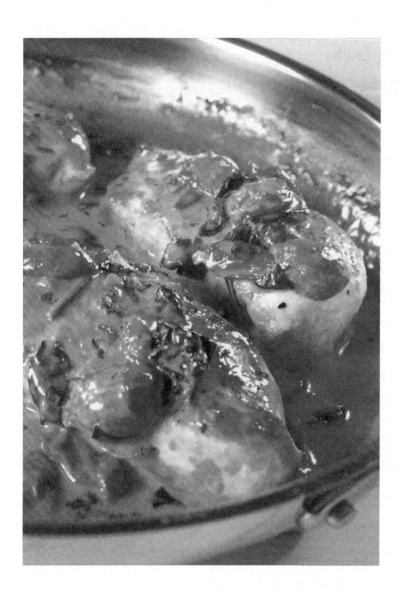

CHICKEN

CREAMY TUSCAN CHICKEN

Weekend family dinner is a momentous occasion by having this creamy dish without making you fat. The stir-fried chicken breast is cooked again in a heavy sauce consisting of plumped cherry tomatoes, Parmesan and heavy cream and drizzled with lemon juice.

Servings: 4

Ingredients

4 **skinless & boneless chicken breasts**

1 tablespoon **extra-virgin olive oil**

Dash of freshly **ground black pepper**

Pinch of **Kosher salt**

3 tablespoons **unsalted butter**

3 minced **cloves garlic**

1 teaspoon **dried oregano**

2 cups **baby spinach**

1 1/2 cups **cherry tomatoes**

1/4 cup freshly grated **Parmesan**

1/2 cup **heavy cream**

Lemon wedges for serving

Directions

Heat olive oil in a large skillet and cook the chicken.

Season with oregano, salt and pepper, flipping once and cook for eight minutes each side until no longer pinkish. Remove chicken from skillet, set aside.

Melt the butter in the same skillet on medium heat.

Stir-fry the garlic for one minute until aromatic.

Stir-fry the cherry tomatoes, season with pepper and salt and cook until the tomatoes are plump.

Stir in spinach until it starts to wilt. Pour the heavy cream and Parmesan cheese; simmer on low heat for three minutes until the sauce has reduced.

Put the chicken to the skillet and cook for five to seven minutes until thoroughly heated.

Remove skillet from stove. Squeeze out the lemon juice from fruit and serve chicken immediately.

Enjoy!

Nutritional Information: 704 calorie; 27 g fat (11.5 g saturated fat); 313 mg cholesterol; 551 mg sodium; 5.3 g carbohydrate; 1.4 g dietary fiber; 2 g total sugars; 110.1 g protein.

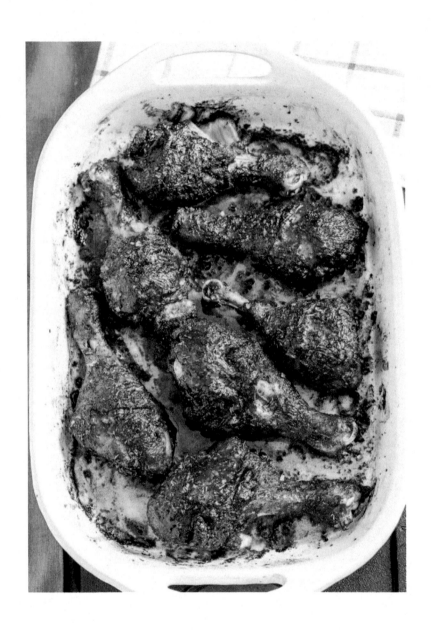

Jerk Chicken

This tender-juicy chicken marinated overnight with a smooth mixture of spices, lemon juice, herbs, sugar, and green onions adds excitement to your outdoor activity. While grilling, the chicken is brushed in the reserved marinade and garnished later with thinly sliced green onions.

Servings: 4

Ingredients

For the chicken:

8 pieces **bone-in chicken drumsticks and thighs**

1 pound bunch **green onions**

2 cloves **garlic**

1 roughly chopped **jalapeno**

Juice of 1 lime

1 tablespoon **light brown sugar**

2 tablespoons **extra-virgin olive oil**

1 teaspoon **dried thyme**

1 1/2 teaspoons **ground allspice**

Kosher salt

1/2 teaspoon **ground cinnamon**

Vegetable oil, for grill

Thinly sliced **green onions** for garnish

Directions

Combine in a blender the green onions, jalapeño, lime juice, garlic, brown sugar, thyme, allspice, olive oil, 2 tablespoons water, 1 teaspoon salt and cinnamon.

Blend the mixture until smooth, setting aside one-fourth cup.

Place the chicken pieces in a shallow dish; sprinkle with salt.

Pour the remaining marinade all over the chicken, tossing to coat well.

Marinate chicken in the fridge for two hours or overnight, turning once in a while to absorb the marinade.

Heat grill on moderate high, and coat grates with oil. Grill the chicken, flipping frequently for ten minutes until charred in spots.

Transfer the grilled chicken few inches away from the hot grill.

Brush with the reserved ¼ cup of marinade. Return to hot grill, cover and cook for additional 10 to 15 minutes until the chicken is cooked thoroughly.

Garnish chicken with green onions.

Enjoy!

Nutritional Information: 743 calorie; 52.5 g fat (13.7 g saturated fat); 285 mg cholesterol; 312 mg sodium; 6.1 g carbohydrate; 1.2 g dietary fiber; 2.9 g total sugars; 63.3 g protein.

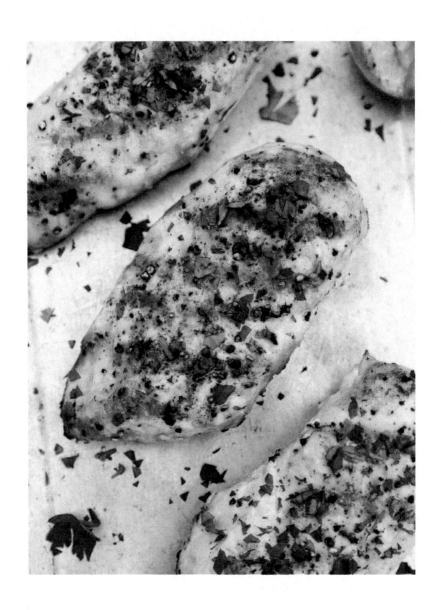

Best Grilled Chicken Breast

The name of this recipe speaks how this grilled chicken breast fare with other grilled meat. The secret is the marinade, which is composed of balsamic vinegar, brown sugar, rosemary, thyme, garlic and black pepper. Its desired taste could be better achieved if you marinate it overnight.

Servings: 4

Ingredients

4 **chicken breasts**

3 tablespoons **extra-virgin olive oil**

1/4 cup **balsamic vinegar**

3 minced **cloves garlic**

2 tablespoons **brown sugar**

1 teaspoon **dried rosemary**

1 teaspoon **dried thyme**

Kosher salt

Freshly ground black pepper

For garnish:

Freshly chopped **parsley**

Directions

Whisk in a medium bowl the olive oil, balsamic vinegar, dried herbs, garlic, and brown sugar.

Season the mixture with generous amount of salt and pepper, reserving one-fourth cup.

Toss the chicken in the marinade and refrigerate for twenty minutes if you are in a hurry or overnight for make ahead.

Preheat the grill to moderate high and grill the marinated chicken.

Baste the reserved ¼ cup marinade and cook for six minutes each side.

Garnish chicken with parsley. Serve warm.

Enjoy!

Nutritional Information: 499 calorie; 19 g fat (1.5 g saturated fat); 215 mg cholesterol; 214 mg sodium; 5.8 g carbohydrate; 0.4 g dietary fiber; 4.5 g total sugars; 71.5 g protein.

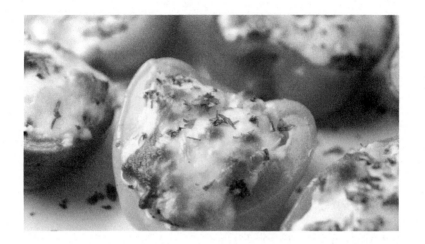

SPINACH ARTICHOKE STUFFED PEPPERS

Each bell pepper is stuffed with chicken mixture consisting of mozzarella, cream cheese, parmesan, garlic, mayo, sour cream, artichoke hearts, rotisserie chicken, and spinach. Every bite of these baked bell peppers is always a pleasure with its creaminess and crunchiness.

Servings: 4-6

Ingredients

Extra-virgin olive oil, for drizzling

4 assorted **bell peppers** (orange, yellow, red & green)

Freshly **ground black pepper**

Pinch of **kosher salt**

1 (14 ounces) can drained and chopped **artichoke hearts**

2 cups shredded **rotisserie chicken**

1 (10 ounces) package thawed, well drained & chopped **spinach**

1 1/2 cups **shredded mozzarella**, divided

6 ounces softened **cream cheese**

1/4 cup **sour cream**

1/2 cup grated **Parmesan**

2 minced **cloves garlic**

1/4 cup **mayonnaise**

Chopped **fresh parsley** for garnish

Directions

Cut into halve the bell peppers and remove the seeds.

Preheat oven at 400° Fahrenheit.

Place the bell peppers on a work surface with cut-side up.

Drizzle with olive oil and sprinkle with salt and pepper.

Combine in a large bowl the shredded rotisserie chicken, spinach, artichoke hearts, ½ cup mozzarella, parmesan cheese, cream cheese, garlic, mayo and sour cream; season with pepper and salt and toss to combine well.

Equally divide the chicken mixture among the pepper halves.

Spread each top with the remaining 1 cup mozzarella cheese.

Bake for twenty-five minutes until the peppers are tender-crisp and the cheese has melted.

Garnish each top with parsley. Serve warm.

Enjoy!

Nutritional Information: 551 calorie; 44.4 g fat (24.4 g saturated fat); 144 mg cholesterol; 728 mg sodium; 20.4 carbohydrate; 5.1 g dietary fiber; 5.7 g total sugars; 23 g protein.

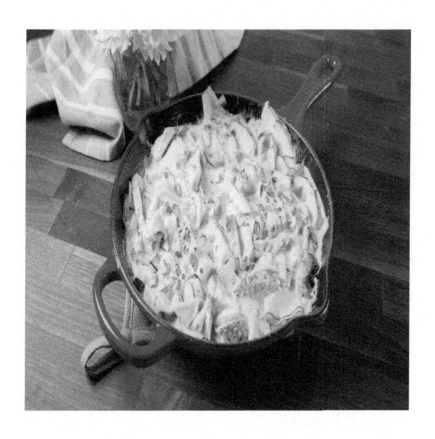

Chicken Zucchini Alfredo

Your desire to stay fit and trim cannot stop you from enjoying this creamy chicken dish with a fake Pappardelle. The pasta is made of zucchini by cutting into long flat, thin strips and cooked together with chicken breasts, Italian seasoning, half-and-half, Parmesan and cream cheese.

Servings: 4

Ingredients

3 large **zucchini**

3/4 pounds **chicken breast**

2 tablespoons **extra-virgin olive oil**, divided

Freshly **ground black pepper**

Kosher salt

4 ounces **cream cheese**

1 teaspoon **Italian seasoning**

3/4 cup **half-and-half or whole milk**

2 finely minced **cloves garlic**

1/2 cup freshly **grated Parmesan**

Additional **grated Parmesan** for serving

1/4 cup fresh chopped **parsley**

Directions

Turn zucchini into Pappardelle or a flat pasta by using a vegetable peeler. Peel into lengthwise to form long and thin strips.

Now place the Pappardelle flat on a baking sheet lined with paper towel, let it stay until ready to use.

Heat 1 tablespoon of olive oil in a large skillet on moderate heat.

Rub each side of chicken breasts with salt, Italian seasoning, and black pepper.

Cook chicken in hot oil for six to eight minutes each side until thoroughly cooked.

Remove from heat and transfer to a cutting board. Slice chicken into thin strips.

Heat the remaining 1 tablespoon of olive oil in the skillet. Stir-fry the garlic for 1 minute until aromatic.

Pour the cream cheese and half-and-half, stirring and cook until the cheese incorporates in the mixture.

Stir in Parmesan, salt and pepper; simmer on low heat for three to five minutes until the sauce is consistent.

Fold in chicken breast with zucchini Pappardelle and chopped parsley. Serve warm.

Enjoy!

Nutritional Information: 451 calorie; 31.1 g fat (14.6 g saturated fat); 123 mg cholesterol; 472 mg sodium; 12.7 g carbohydrate; 2.8 g dietary fiber; 4.5 g total sugars; 33.7 g protein.

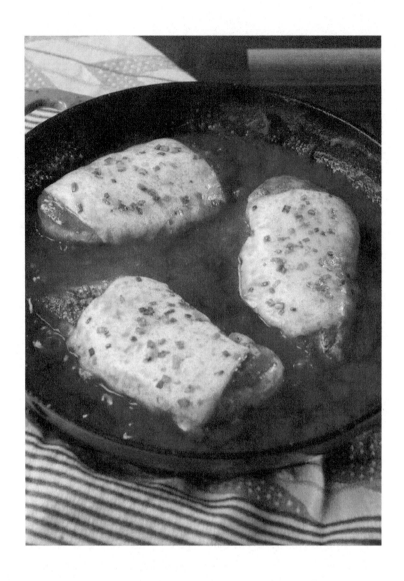

Buffalo Skillet Chicken

Picky eaters will love these delightful chicken skillets in oil before mixing with the buffalo sauce in butter mixture. Each chicken breast is topped with two slices of Muenster that add a cheesy flavor, which is appealing to your taste buds.

Servings: 4

Ingredients

4 **boneless skinless chicken breasts**

Kosher salt

1 teaspoon **garlic powder**

1 tablespoon **extra-virgin olive oil**

2 tablespoons **butter**

Freshly **ground black pepper**

Pinch of **cayenne pepper**

1 cup **buffalo sauce**

2 minced **cloves garlic**

8 slices of **Muenster**

For garnish:

Fresh chopped **chives**

Directions

Heat olive oil in a large skillet on medium heat.

Cook the chicken breast in hot oil for six minutes each side; season with pepper, garlic powder and salt.

Place cooked chicken on a plate. In the same skillet, melt the butter and cook the garlic for 1 minute until fragrant.

Stir in buffalo sauce and cayenne.

Place the chicken in the skillet, topping each breast with two slices of Muenster cheese.

Cover the skillet and simmer the chicken on low heat for three minutes or more.

When done, garnish on top with chives. Serve chicken with greens.

Enjoy!

Nutritional Information: 785 calorie; 32.1 g fat (14.9 g saturated fat); 329 mg cholesterol; 1692 mg sodium; 3.7 g carbohydrate; 1.1 g dietary fiber; 0.8 g total sugars; 117.4 g protein.

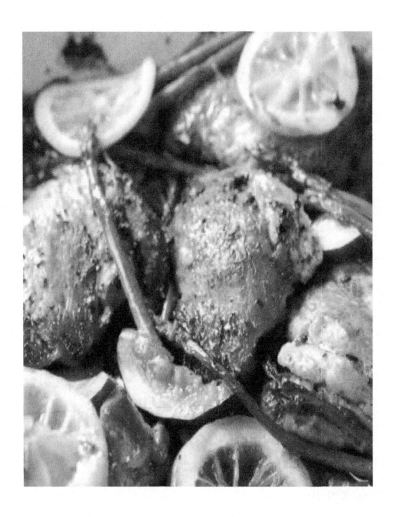

GARLICKY GREEK CHICKEN

Marinating the chicken with a mixture of lemon juice, oregano, olive oil and garlic is the secret of its flavorful and tangy taste. The chicken is seared before mixing with asparagus, lemons and zucchini and then baked in the oven for a crusty texture.

Servings: 4

Ingredients

Juice of 1 lemon

3 tablespoons **extra-virgin olive oil**, divided

1 teaspoon **dried oregano**

3 minced **cloves garlic**

Pinch **kosher salt**

1 pound **chicken thighs**

1/2 pound **asparagus** (remove the ends)

Freshly **ground black pepper**

1 sliced into **half-moons zucchini**

1 sliced **lemon**

Directions

Combine in a large bowl the lemon juice, oregano, 2 tablespoons of olive oil and garlic, whisking until incorporated. Toss chicken thighs and toss to coat with mixture.

Cover the bowl with a plastic wrap and marinate the chicken for fifteen minutes to two hours in the refrigerator.

Preheat oven at 425 degrees F.

76

Heat the remaining 1 tablespoon of olive oil in an ovenproof pan on medium heat.

Remove marinated chicken and season both sides with salt and pepper.

Place the chicken in pan with skin-side facing down and pour the marinade all over.

Sear the chicken for ten minutes until crisp-golden. Turn chicken once to cook the other side and stir in asparagus, lemons and zucchini half-moon slices.

Place the pan in the oven and cook the chicken for fifteen minutes.

Remove chicken when done and the veggies are tender-crisp.

Enjoy!

Nutritional Information: 333 calorie; 19.2 g fat (3.9 g saturated fat); 101 mg cholesterol; 143 mg sodium; 6.2 g carbohydrate; 2.4 g dietary fiber; 2.3 g total sugars; 35 g protein.

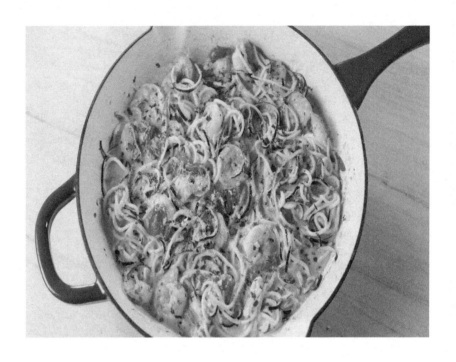

Shrimp

Garlicky Shrimp Zucchini Pasta

You love pasta, but you're on a diet program, what else is the best option to enjoy pasta without feeling guilty. Try spiralized zucchini pasta and add it to your creamy-garlicky shrimp dish. You've got to enjoy every bite of this awesome pasta alternative.

Servings: 3-4

Ingredients

1 pound peeled and deveined medium or large **shrimp**

3 tablespoons **butter**, divided

Freshly **ground black pepper**

Kosher salt

3/4 cup **heavy cream**

3 minced **cloves garlic**

1 cup halved **cherry tomatoes**

1/2 cup grated **Parmesan**

3 tablespoons large **zucchini** (spiralized)

3 tablespoons freshly chopped **parsley**

Directions

Melt 1 tablespoon of butter in a large skillet on moderate heat.

Stir-fry the shrimp and sprinkle with a pinch of salt and pepper. Cook for two minutes each side until the shrimp is pinkish in color.

Place cooked shrimp on a platter and the juices remain in the skillet.

Melt the remaining 2 tablespoons of butter and sauté the garlic for 1 minute until fragrant.

Whisk in the heavy cream, simmer and stir in tomato halves, parsley and Parmesan.

Simmer mixture until the vegetables are soft and the sauce is slightly consistent for three minutes.

Place the shrimp in the skillet with the zucchini noodles, tossing to combine well.

Enjoy!

Nutritional Information: 359 calorie; 25.1 g fat (15.7 g saturated fat); 205 mg cholesterol; 1167 mg sodium; 5.6 g carbohydrate; 1.4 g total sugars; 0.8 g dietary fiber; 31.5 g protein.

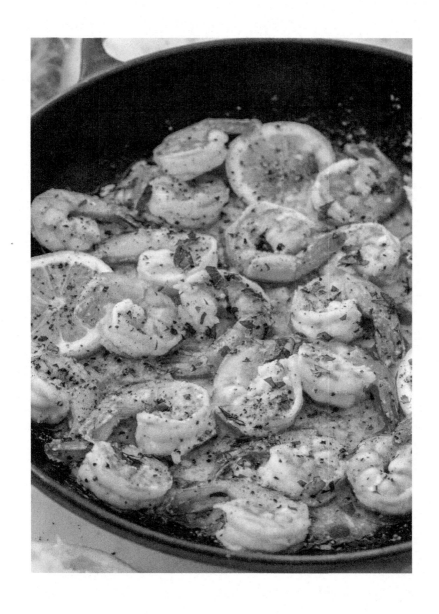

Lemon Garlic Shrimp

This shrimp recipe is perhaps the easiest and can be finished in 20 minutes. Sauté the shrimp in melted butter and oil, together with garlic and red pepper flakes. Adding more flavors to the shrimp is the white wine, more butter, and parsley and lemon juice.

Servings: 4

Ingredients

1 pound peeled and deveined medium **shrimp**

1 tablespoon **extra-virgin olive oil**

2 tablespoons **butter**, divided

3 minced **cloves garlic**

Juice of 1 lemon

1 teaspoon crushed **red pepper flakes**

2 tablespoons **dry white wine**

For garnish:

Freshly chopped **parsley**

Directions

Melt one tablespoon of butter together with olive oil in a large skillet on moderate heat.

Sauté the shrimp, crushed red pepper flakes and garlic for three minutes until the shrimp changes color to pink.

Remove skillet from heat and stir in lemon juice, parsley, white wine and 1 tablespoon of butter.

Serve!

Nutritional Information: 232 calorie; 11.3 g fat (4.8 g saturated fat); 254 mg cholesterol; 320 mg sodium; 4.4 g carbohydrate; 0.7 g dietary fiber; 0.5 g total sugars; 26.3 g protein.

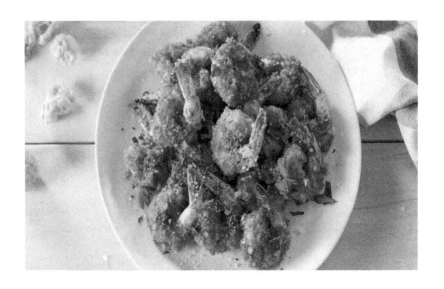

BREADED SHRIMP

Breaded shrimp is a favorite food in family reunions, but if you are on a diet, this recipe is given a twist by not using flour in coating the shrimp, instead it makes use of pork rind mixture consisting of garlic powder, oregano, Parmesan, paprika, black pepper, chili powder, and salt.

Servings: 4

Ingredients

6 ounces **pork rinds**

Cooking spray

1/4 cup grated **Parmesan**

1/2 teaspoon **paprika**

1 teaspoon **chili powder**

1/2 teaspoon **dried oregano**

1/2 teaspoon **garlic powder**

Freshly **ground black pepper**

2 beaten large **eggs**

Kosher salt

1 pound large **shrimp**

For the sauce:

Juice of 1/2 lemon

1/2 cup **mayonnaise** or **sour cream**

Dash of **hot sauce**

For garnish:

Freshly chopped **parsley**

Directions

Preheat oven at 450° Fahrenheit. Coat the bottom of a large-sized rimmed baking sheet with cooking spray.

Place pork rinds in a food processor and crush into fine crumbs.

Place crumbs in a shallow bowl, whisk in paprika, parmesan, chili powder, dried oregano, garlic powder, salt and black pepper.

In a shallow bowl, pour the beaten eggs and dredge the shrimp.

Tap excess egg to drip and coat well with pork rind mixture.

Neatly place the breaded shrimp on the baking sheet and bake for ten to twelve minutes until crispy and thoroughly cooked.

Prepare the sauce by whisking the lemon juice, hot sauce and mayonnaise. Garnish the shrimp with parsley.

Serve!

Nutritional Information: 537 calorie; 30.8 g fat (10.4 g saturated fat); 333 mg cholesterol; 1385 mg sodium; 11.3 g carbohydrate; 0.6 g dietary fiber; 2.4 g total sugars; 56.8 g protein.

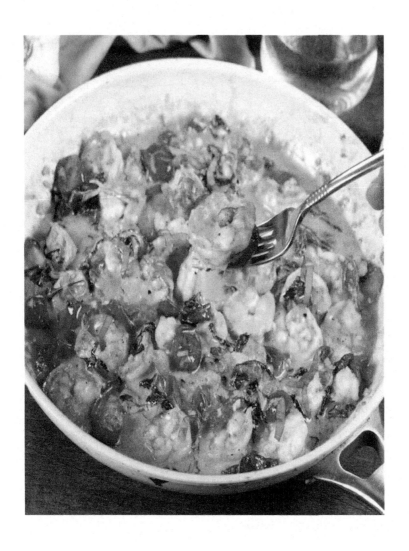

TUSCAN BUTTER SHRIMP

Feel the Tuscan air with this Keto buttered shrimp. The shrimp is seared in shimmering olive oil and cooked with the goodness of heavy cream, Parmesan, basil, tomatoes, spinach and sprinkled with herbs and squeezed with lemon juice.

Servings: 4

Ingredients

1 pound **shrimp**

2 tablespoons **extra-virgin olive oil**

Freshly **ground black pepper**

Pinch of **kosher salt**

3 minced **cloves garlic**

3 tablespoons **unsalted butter**

2 cups **baby spinach**

1 1/2 cup halved **cherry tomatoes**

1/4 cup freshly **grated Parmesan**

1/2 cup **heavy cream**

1/4 cup thinly sliced **basil**

Lemon wedges for serving

Directions

Peel, devein the shrimp and remove the tails; season all over with salt and pepper.

Heat the olive oil in a large pan on medium high heat.

Cook the shrimp in shimmering oil, sear for two minutes and flip once, until its underside turns golden.

Remove shrimp from pan, set aside. Add butter to the pan and melt on medium heat.

Stir-fry garlic for 1 minute until fragrant. Stir in cherry tomatoes, add salt and pepper.

Stir until the tomatoes are starting to burst. Stir in spinach until it starts to wilt.

Pour heavy cream, basil and Parmesan and bring to a simmer.

Cook on low heat and simmer for three minutes until a bit reduced.

Place the shrimp again in the pan and toss to incorporate with the ingredients and cook until heated thoroughly.

Sprinkle with herbs and drizzle with lemon juice.

Return shrimp to skillet and stir to combine.

Cook until shrimp is heated through, garnish with more herbs and squeeze lemon on top before serving.

Enjoy!

Nutritional Information: 387 calorie; 26.3 g fat (12.5 g saturated fat); 292 mg cholesterol; 528 mg sodium; 6.6 g carbohydrate; 1.2 g dietary fiber; 1.9 g total sugars; 31.9 g protein.

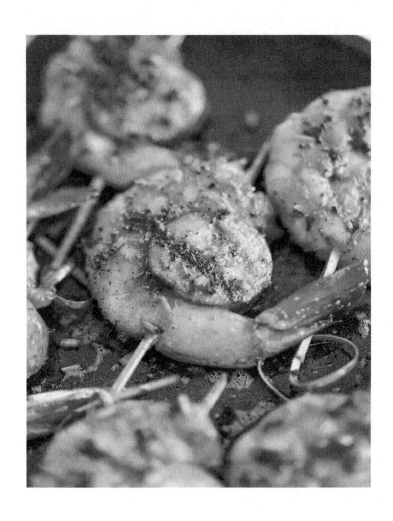

Cajun Shrimp Kebabs

Grilled shrimp is a healthy cooking method rather than fry them in oil. Toss the shrimp in oil and then in the spice mix, which is a blend of salt, paprika, garlic powder, oregano, onion powder, and cayenne. Thread the shrimp and lemon slices before putting on the grill to cook.

Servings: 4-6

Ingredients

1 pound **shrimp**

1 teaspoon **kosher salt**

2 tablespoons **olive oil**

1 teaspoon **cayenne**

1 teaspoon **oregano**

1 teaspoon **paprika**

1 teaspoon **onion powder**

1 teaspoon **garlic powder**

2 thinly sliced **crosswise lemons**

Directions

Preheat grill to moderate high heat.

Combine in a small bowl the salt, paprika, garlic powder, cayenne, and oregano and onion powder, stirring to combine well.

Pour the olive oil in a medium-size bowl and toss the shrimp to coat with oil.

Pour the spice mix in the bowl, tossing the shrimp again until fully coated.

With metal skewers or bamboo skewers, thread the shrimp, lemon, shrimp, lemon, shrimp, lemon and shrimp in this order or if you like it the other way around, whichever you feel more comfortable for you.

Grill skewers for four to five minutes until the lemon is charred and aromatic and the shrimp is opaque in color.

Flip once to cook the other side.

Serve!

Nutritional Information: 212 calorie; 9.2 g fat (1.6 g saturated fat); 239 mg cholesterol; 860 mg sodium; 6.2 g carbohydrate; 1.4 g dietary fiber; 1.2 g total sugars; 26.5 g protein.

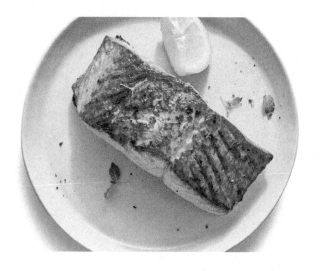

Fish

Broiled Salmon

Dieters prefer to eat fish with carefully chosen ingredients to stay fit, like this Broiled Salmon. The fish is covered with dressing consisting of lemon juice, shallot, rosemary, thyme, mustard, and garlic and seasoned with salt and pepper and no seasonings to enhance its taste, but simply relying on herbs.

Servings: 4

Ingredients

4 (4-ounces) **salmon fillets**

2 finely minced **cloves garlic**

1 tablespoon **Grainy mustard**

2 teaspoons chopped **fresh thyme leaves**

Additional **thyme leaves** for garnish

1 tablespoon finely minced **shallots**

2 teaspoons chopped **fresh rosemary**

Pinch of **kosher salt**

Juice of 1/2 **lemon**

Freshly **ground black pepper**

Slices of lemon for serving

Directions

Preheat the broiler. Prepare a baking sheet by lining with a parchment.

Combine in a small bowl the garlic, mustard, salt, pepper, lemon juice, rosemary, thyme and shallot. Stir and spread over the salmon fillet.

Place in the broiler and broil for seven to eight minutes.

Top salmon with thyme leaves and slices of lemon.

Nutritional Information: 248 calorie; 11.3 g fat (1.6 g saturated fat); 78 mg cholesterol; 135 mg sodium; 2.6 g carbohydrate; 0.7 g dietary fiber; 0.2 g total sugars; 34.9 g protein.

Lemony Grilled Salmon

This grilled fish does not call for seasonings, herbs and tons of spices, except for black pepper, and butter. The fish is brushed with olive oil before grilling and then topped with grilled lemon slices when serving.

Servings: 4

Ingredients

Extra-virgin olive oil for brushing

4 (6-ounces) **skin-on salmon fillets**

Freshly **ground black pepper**

Pinch of **kosher salt**

2 tablespoons **butter**

2 sliced **lemons**

Directions

Heat your grill to high.

Prepare the salmon by brushing with oil, and season with a pinch of salt and pepper.

Place the salmon and slices of lemon on the hot grill.

Cook salmon thoroughly until charred for five minutes each side.

Remove salmon from grill, pat with butter and place on top with grilled lemon.

Enjoy!

Nutritional Information: 590.8 calories, 48 g protein, 4.3 g carbohydrate, 41 g fat (17.7 g saturated), 172.5 mg cholesterol, 468.8 mg sodium.

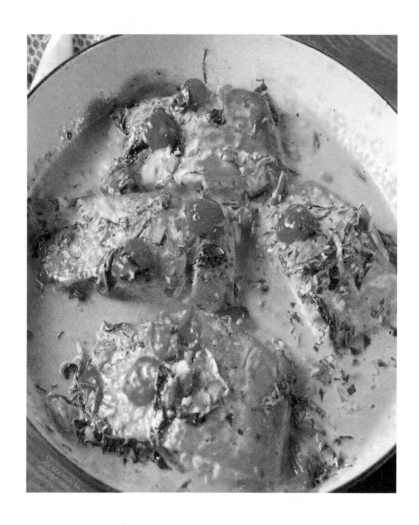

Tuscan Butter Salmon

This recipe is popular in parties because of its simplicity, yet exudes elegance. The salmon is fried first until golden before mixing with the creamy sauce, which is a blend of cherry tomatoes, heavy cream, parmesan, baby spinach, and chopped herbs (basil and parsley).

Servings: 4

Ingredients

2 tablespoons of **extra-virgin olive oil**

Kosher salt

4 (6 ounces) **salmon fillets**

Freshly **ground black pepper**

3 tablespoons **butter**

1 1/2 cups halved **cherry tomatoes**

3 minced **cloves garlic**

1/2 cup **heavy cream**

2 cups **baby spinach**

1/4 cup freshly grated **Parmesan**

1/4 cup chopped **herbs** (ex: basil and parsley)

Additional **herbs** for garnish

Lemon wedges for serving

Directions

Pat dry salmon fillets with paper towels and season all over with pepper and salt.

Heat 2 tablespoons of olive oil in a large-sized skillet on medium high heat.

Cook the salmon with skin-side up in shimmering oil for six minutes until deep golden.

Flip and cook for two minutes each side.

Place cooked salmon on a plate. Heat the butter in the same skillet over moderate heat until melted.

Stir-fry the garlic for 1 minute until fragrant.

Sauté cherry tomatoes and sprinkle with salt and pepper; cook until the tomatoes start to burst.

Stir in spinach and cook until it starts to wilt.

Pour heavy cream, chopped herbs and Parmesan; simmer on low heat for three minutes until the sauce has reduced. Place the salmon in the skillet.

Spoon the sauce over salmon; simmer for three minutes until thoroughly cooked.

Garnish salmon with additional chopped herbs and squeeze out lemon on top.

Enjoy!

Nutritional Information: 482 calorie; 35 g fat (13.5 g saturated fat); 128 mg cholesterol; 327 mg sodium; 6.1 g carbohydrate; 2.1 g dietary fiber; 1.9 g total sugars; 39.4 g protein.

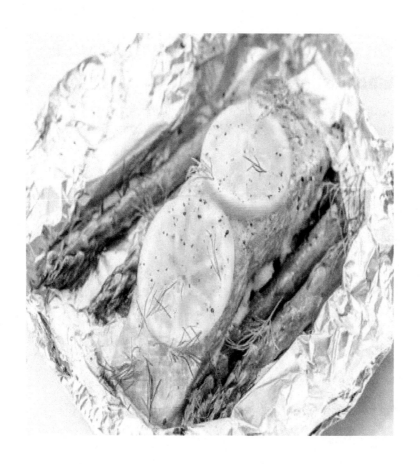

Foil Pack Grilled Salmon with Lemony Asparagus

Dieters will surely embrace this method of preparing fish because of its simplicity and tangy aroma. All you have to do is to lay the asparagus on foil and top with asparagus, butter and lemon slices with salt and pepper. Fold the foil and grill.

Servings: 4

Ingredients

20 trimmed **asparagus spears**

4 (6 ounces) **skin-on salmon fillets**

2 sliced **lemons**

4 tablespoons **butter**, divided

Dash of freshly **ground black pepper**

Pinch of **kosher salt**

For garnish:

Torn **fresh dill**

Directions

Place 2 aluminum foils on a flat work surface and place on top, 5 asparagus spears.

Place on top of asparagus the salmon fillet, one tablespoon of butter and 2 lemon slices; sprinkle with salt and pepper.

Wrap by folding the edges to the center.

Repeat with the rest of the asparagus, salmon fillet, butter and lemon slices to come up with 4 packets.

Preheat grill and place the four packets on baking sheet until the fish is thoroughly cooked and the asparagus is tender-crisp for ten minutes.

Garnish salmon with torn dill.

Serve!

Nutritional Information: 414 calorie; 26.3 g fat (9.8 g saturated fat); 134 mg cholesterol; 122 mg sodium; 7.4 g carbohydrate; 3.3 g dietary fiber; 3 g total sugars; 39.5 g protein.

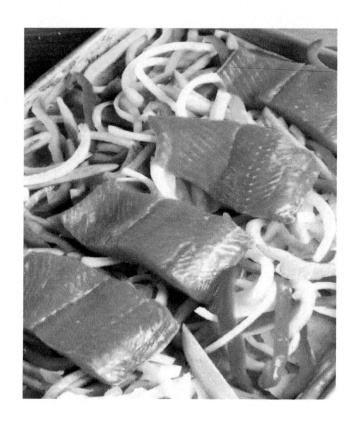

BAKED CAJUN SALMON

Baked salmon with myriads of herbs, spices and Cajun seasoning cooked together in one sitting will result an elegant and aromatic dish. It is not only appealing to look at, but the method is very simple. After preparing the ingredients, put them together in a baking sheet and bake for a few minutes.

Servings: 4

Ingredients

1 thinly sliced **red bell pepper**

1/2 thinly sliced large **white onion**

3 thinly sliced **cloves garlic**

1 thinly sliced **orange bell pepper**

Freshly **ground black pepper**

Pinch of **kosher salt**

1 tablespoon **dried thyme**

3 tablespoons **extra-virgin olive oil**

2 teaspoon **paprika**

1 tablespoon **Cajun seasoning**

2 teaspoon **garlic powder**

4 pieces (6 ounces) **salmon fillets**

Directions

Preheat oven at 400° Fahrenheit.

Prepare a large baking sheet and place the thinly sliced onions, garlic and peppers and sprinkle with salt and pepper; toss with olive oil.

Meanwhile, prepare the seasoning blend in a small bowl by whisking the Cajun seasoning, garlic powder, paprika and thyme.

Place the salmon fillets on the baking sheet lined with herbs.

Spread on top of salmon the seasoning blend, rubbing all over the fillets.

Bake for twenty minutes until the salmon is thoroughly cooked and the veggies are tender.

Enjoy!

Nutritional Information: 188 calorie; 13.6 g fat (1.9 g saturated fat); 20 mg cholesterol; 100 mg sodium; 9.1 g carbohydrate; 2 g dietary fiber; 4.3 g total sugars; 10.1 g protein.

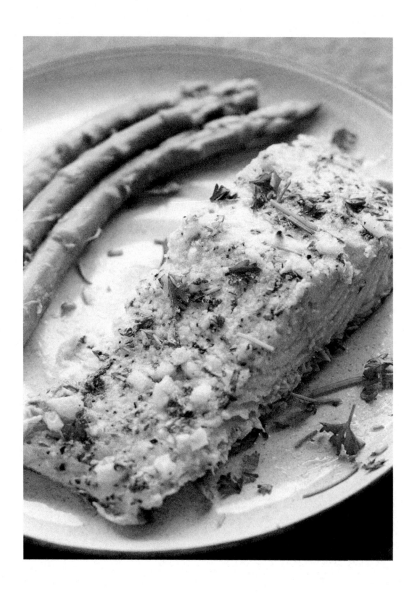

Garlic Parmesan Salmon

Bring out the flavor of your baked salmon by brushing with garlic mixture, which is a combination of olive oil, parsley, salt, pepper, Parmesan and garlic. When serving, garnish the salmon with grated Parmesan cheese.

Servings: 6

Ingredients

1 tablespoon of **extra-virgin olive oil**

1 (2-3 pounds) **salmon fillet**

2 tablespoons freshly chopped **parsley**

1/4 cup finely grated **Parmesan**

4 minced **cloves garlic**

Pinch of **Kosher salt**

Dash of freshly **ground black pepper**

Directions

Preheat oven at 400 degrees F and coat a piece of aluminum foil with cooking spray.

Combine together in a small bowl the olive oil, Parmesan, garlic, parsley, salt and pepper, stir to incorporate.

Place the foil on top of a large rimmed baking sheet and put the salmon on top of foil.

Brush salmon with garlic mixture and cover with foil.

Bake for fifteen to twenty minutes until cooked thoroughly.

Garnish with grated Parmesan.

Serve!

Nutritional Information: 353 calorie; 18.4 g fat (3.7 g saturated fat); 107 mg cholesterol; 215 mg sodium; 1.1 g carbohydrate; 0.1 g dietary fiber; 0 g total sugars; 47.2 g protein.

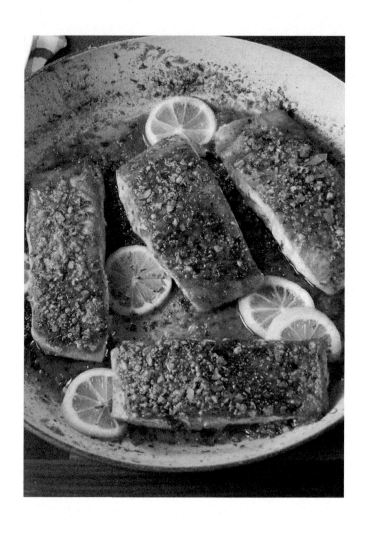

Cajun Parmesan Salmon

This recipe calls for wild salmon for a much better taste, but if you can't find, it does not matter if you use salmon fillets. The salmon is seasoned with Cajun seasoning before frying and then cooked with a thick sauce consisting of honey, chicken broth, lemon juice, Cajun seasoning, spices and Parmesan.

Servings: 4

Ingredients

4 (4 ounces) **fillets salmon**

1 tablespoon **extra-virgin olive oil**

Freshly **ground black pepper**

2 teaspoons **Cajun seasoning**

2 tablespoons **butter**

1/3 cup **low-sodium chicken** or **vegetable broth**

3 cloves minced **garlic**

1 tablespoon **honey**

Juice of 1 lemon

1 tablespoon freshly chopped **parsley**

2 tablespoons freshly grated **Parmesan**

Additional chopped **parsley** for garnish

Lemon slices for serving

Directions

Heat olive oil in a large frying pan over medium high heat.

Season the salmon with dash of pepper and one teaspoon Cajun seasoning.

Cook salmon in hot oil with skin-side up for six minutes until golden brown; turn once and cook the other side for 2 minutes. Transfer salmon on paper towels.

Melt the butter in the pan and cook the garlic.

Stir in lemon juice, chicken or vegetable broth, honey, parsley, Parmesan and the remaining 1 teaspoon Cajun seasoning; bring to a simmer.

Continue cooking on medium heat and return the salmon to the pan; simmer for three to four minutes until the fish is cooked and the sauce is consistent.

Place lemon slices on top of salmon.

Serve!

Nutritional Information: 391 calorie; 21.9 g fat (7.7 g saturated fat); 54 mg cholesterol; 247 mg sodium; 6.7 g carbohydrate; 0.6 g dietary fiber; 4.8 g total sugars; 42.9 g protein.

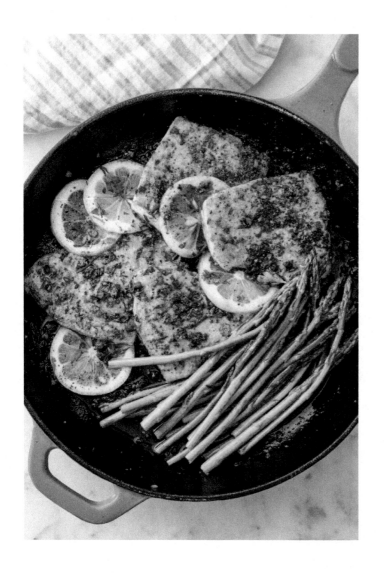

GARLICKY LEMON MAHI MAHI

Prepare a delicious fish dish in 25 minutes only. It is an easy recipe for the lazy you. The fish fillet is cooked with butter and olive oil and then cooked again in lemony sauce with chopped parsley. It is a perfect treat for weight watchers.

Servings: 4

Ingredients

1 tablespoon **extra-virgin olive oil**

3 tablespoons **butter**, divided

4 (4 ounces) **mahi-mahi fillets**

Freshly **ground black pepper**

Pinch of **kosher salt**

Juice and zest of 1 lemon

3 minced **cloves garlic**

1 tablespoon freshly chopped **parsley**

Additional chopped **parsley** for garnish

Directions

Melt one tablespoon of butter with olive oil in a large pan on medium heat.

Place mahi mahi fillet in the pan and sprinkle with a pinch of salt and pepper.

Cook the fish for three minutes each side until golden and transfer into a plate.

114

Heat the remaining two tablespoons of butter in skillet and cook the garlic for 1 minute until fragrant.

Stir in parsley, and juice and zest of 1 lemon. Place the fish fillet in the skillet and spoon the sauce to cover.

Garnish fish with additional chopped parsley.

Enjoy!

Nutritional Information: 204 calorie; 12.2 g fat (6 g saturated fat); 63 mg cholesterol; 196 mg sodium; 2.2 g carbohydrate; 0.5 g dietary fiber; 0.4 g total sugars; 21.4 g protein.

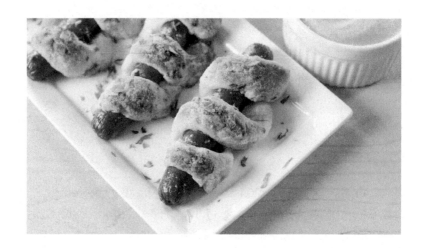

116

HOTDOG

KETO DOGS

Enjoy your snacks even if you are on a diet by preparing these adorable hot dogs wrapped in homemade rope dough. Use almond flour with baking powder, salt, and eggs when making the dough and brush all over with a mixture of garlic powder, butter and parsley. Bake hotdog with rope together.

Servings: 6

Ingredients

8 **hot dogs**

4 ounces **cream cheese**

2 cups shredded **mozzarella**

2 1/2 cups **almond flour**

2 beaten large **eggs**

1 teaspoon **kosher salt**

2 teaspoons **baking powder**

1 tablespoon freshly chopped **parsley**

4 tablespoons melted **butter**

1 teaspoon **garlic powder**

Mustard for serving

Directions

Preheat oven at 400° F, and line your baking sheet with a parchment paper.

In a heat-proof bowl, melt both cream cheese and mozzarella cheese.

Stir in eggs and add the baking powder, salt, and almond flour.

Divide the dough into eight ball pieces and form them into long ropes.

Wrap around the dough rope around individual hotdogs.

Whisk in a small bowl the parsley, garlic powder and butter and then brush over the hot dog and dough rope.

Bake for ten to fifteen minutes until golden. Serve dogs with mustard.

Enjoy!

Nutritional Information: 577 calorie; 42.3 g fat (17.6 g saturated fat); 141 mg cholesterol: 1553 mg sodium; 30.2 g carbohydrate; 2.8 g dietary fiber; 6.1 g total sugars; 21 g protein.

Bacon

Bacon Wrapped Stuffed Zucchini

Love these zucchini boats stuffed with creamy vegetable mixture and wrapped with bacon slices. It's spicy and creamy taste are its plus factor why dieters prefer this. Spoon out the seedy flesh of the zucchini and fill with stuffing before placing in the oven.

Servings: 6

Ingredients

3 medium **zucchini**, cut into half lengthwise

1/2 cup finely chopped **artichoke hearts**

8 ounces softened **cream cheese**

1 cup shredded **mozzarella**

1/2 cup frozen **spinach**

1/2 cup freshly grated **Parmesan**

1/2 teaspoon **red pepper flakes**

Extra **red pepper flakes** for garnish

1 minced **garlic clove**

Freshly **ground black pepper**

Pinch of **kosher salt**

12 slices of **bacon**

Directions

Defrost, drain and chop frozen spinach, set aside.

Preheat oven at 350° F. Fit a parchment paper-lined baking sheet with a cooling rack.

Scoop out the flesh from the seedy center of zucchini.

Mix altogether in a large bowl the artichoke hearts, cream cheese, red pepper flakes, garlic, spinach, mozzarella, and Parmesan.

Sprinkle mixture with salt and pepper, toss to combine well.

Fill each zucchini boat with cream cheese mixture and wrap 2 slices of bacon around each boat.

Place zucchini boats on cooling rack and bake for thirty-five to forty minutes until the bacon and zucchini are both crisp-tender.

Slightly cool and serve.

Enjoy!

Nutritional Information: 418 calorie; 33.1 g fat (16.1 g saturated fat); 96 mg cholesterol; 1217 mg sodium; 5.3 g carbohydrate; 1.2 g dietary fiber; 1.8 g total sugars; 23.6 g protein.

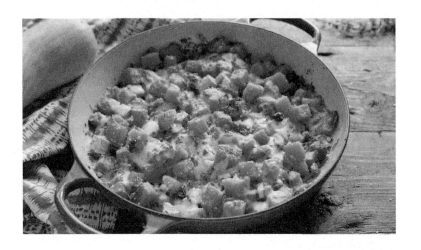

CHEESY BACON BUTTERNUT SQUASH

This baked butternut squash is packed with herbs, bacon and cheeses that add more appeal to your taste buds. Once tasted, non-vegans will surely like the squash without any qualms, a great way to stay fit and enjoying a hearty meal.

Servings: 6

Ingredients

2 pounds **butternut squash**

2 minced **cloves garlic**

2 tablespoons **olive oil**

Kosher salt

2 tablespoons chopped **thyme**

1/2 pound chopped **bacon**

Freshly **ground black pepper**

1/2 cup freshly grated **Parmesan**

1 1/2 cup shredded **mozzarella**

Garnish:

Chopped **fresh parsley**

Directions

Peel and cut butternut squash into one-inch pieces.

Preheat oven at 425° Fahrenheit. Toss cubed butternut squash in a large baking dish.

Sprinkle squash with olive oil, salt, pepper; add the garlic and thyme.

Spread the cubed bacon on top of squash.

Bake butternut squash for twenty to twenty-five minutes until tender and the bacon is crisp.

Remove baking dish from oven and garnish squash with cheeses.

Return to oven and bake for five to ten minutes until the cheeses have melted. Sprinkle with parsley.

Serve!

Nutritional Information: 397 calorie; 26 g fat (9.3 g saturated fat); 59 mg cholesterol; 1124 mg sodium; 20.2 g carbohydrate; 3.4 g dietary fiber; 3.4 g total sugars.

Bacon Avocado Bombs

There are only three ingredients required for these delicious avocado bombs. Peel the skin of the avocado and remove the pit, peel the avocado with shredded cheese and cover with the other half without cheese. Cover the avocado with slices of bacon and broil.

Servings: 4

Ingredients

2 **avocados**

8 slices **bacon**

1/3 cup shredded **Cheddar**

Directions

Heat the broiler and line a small baking sheet with aluminum tin foil.

Slice the avocado in half and discard the pit.

Remove the skin of the avocado and stuff each two avocado halves with shredded cheese and replace with the other avocado halves without cheese.

Wrap the avocado half with four bacon slices.

Place on the baking sheet; broil until the bacon is crispy for five minutes, flipping with tongs and continue cooking until crispy for five minutes each side.

Cut the broiled avocado into half crosswise, serve warm.

Serve!

Nutritional Information: 427 calorie; 36.1 g fat (9.8 g saturated fat); 44 mg cholesterol; 941 mg sodium; 9.4 g carbohydrate; 6.7 g dietary fiber; 0.6 g total sugars; 18.3 g protein.

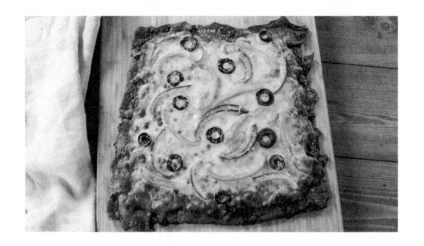

Bacon Weave Pizza

Imagine having a pizza made of crusty bacon, and not the usual flour-based crust. It is not only a weight loss recommended diet, but the pizza tastes yummier, meatier and saucy. This recipe is effortless as you don't have to spend time in preparing the dough.

Serving: 1 pizza (4 slices)

Ingredients

12 slices **thick-cut bacon**

1 cup shredded **mozzarella**

1/2 cup **pizza sauce**

1/4 sliced medium **red onion**

1 cup sliced **green bell pepper**

1/4 cup grated **Parmesan**

1/4 cup sliced **black olives**

Directions

Preheat oven at 400° Fahrenheit.

Prepare a large baking sheet by lining with parchment paper.

Prepare the bacon by lining six slices side-by-side on your baking sheet, lifting up and folding back every other slice and place the 7th slice on top in the middle part.

Lay the folded-back bacon slices on top of the 7th slice, folding back the alternate bacon slice. Place the 8th bacon slice on the top right, next to the 7th bacon slice.

Repeat the weaving steps four times to come up with four pizza slices later.

Put on top of the bacon weaves a heat-proof cooling rack in an inverted position to keep the bacon stay flat instead of curling when baking.

Bake the bacon weaves for twenty-three to twenty-five minutes until crisps. Remove the baking sheet from oven and drain excess fat.

Slowly lift the inverted cooling rack. Spread on top of bacon weaves the pizza sauce with at least ½-inch allowance for the crust.

Garnish with mozzarella cheese, pepper, olives, onions and Parmesan cheese.

Place the baking sheet back in the oven and bake for ten minutes more until the cheese becomes melty.

Serve!

Nutritional Information: 271 calorie; 19 g fat (7 g saturated fat); 42 mg cholesterol; 809 mg sodium; 7.2 g carbohydrate; 1.3 g dietary fiber; 2.8 g total sugars; 15.1 g protein.

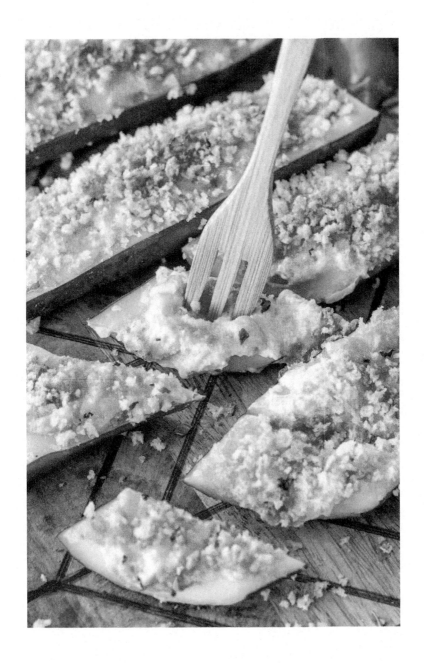

Jalapeño Popper Stuffed Zucchini

There are many ways to enjoy a jalapeno, without detecting its hot taste. Make it as part of your filling for your zucchini slices. Mix the cream cheese, jalapeño, garlic powder, cheddar, bacon and ½ cup mozzarella to create the popper filling and place them in between slices of zucchini.

Servings: 6

Ingredients

6 ounces softened **cream cheese**

3 **zucchini** cut into half crosswise

1/2 cup **shredded Cheddar**

1 cup **shredded mozzarella**, divided

4 slices **cooked and crumbled bacon**

1 tablespoon **cooked and crumbled bacon** for topping

1 teaspoon **garlic powder**

1 minced **jalapeno**

Freshly **ground black pepper**

1 tablespoon chopped **parsley**

Kosher salt

Directions

Preheat the oven at 425° F.

Cut the top ends of each zucchini and discard.

Slice the rest of the zucchini with skin on, about one-fourth inch pieces on top of chopsticks.

Place sliced zucchini on a rimmed baking sheet lined with a parchment. Bake for ten minutes until pliable.

Prepare the jalapeño popper filling by combining in a medium-size bowl the cream cheese, jalapeño, garlic powder, cheddar, bacon and ½ cup mozzarella.

Season the filling with salt and pepper; stir to combine well. Remove baked zucchini from oven.

Stuff the zucchini between each slice with jalapeño mixture.

Sprinkle bacon and mozzarella on top of each zucchini. Bake zucchini again for six to eight minutes, until the cheese has melted.

Scatter on top with parsley.

Serve!

Nutritional Information: 215 calorie; 16.9 g fat (8.9 g saturated fat); 50 mg cholesterol; 500 mg sodium; 5.1 g carbohydrate; 1.2 g dietary fiber; 2 g total sugars; 11.8 g protein.

CONCLUSION

Thank you so much for purchasing this book. We at Savour Press hope this book has increased your knowledge regarding some unique recipes. This Book contains a curated list of what we believe to be the best recipes to manage and treat gestational diabetes which cover a variety of cooking methods, flavors, and tastes. All different categories of foods are represented such as your beef, pork, pasta, chicken, fish bacon , shrimp , and among others.

During the creation of this cookbook, we made sure that every ingredient should be easily accessible, and that the recipes are presented in such a way that they are understandable in layman's language. We are aware of your desire to stay fit and in your top form, and this we come up with our edition of Keto Diet cookbook, to give you lots of recipe choices so every meal is always a pleasurable occasion. We hope you will enjoy cooking with these recipes.

Thanks again for your support.

Happy Cooking!

Printed in Great Britain
by Amazon

41661521R00076